The Ultimate Keto Slow Cooker Recipe Collection

50 Tasty and Affordable Keto Recipes to Delight Your Day with the Right Foot

Katherine Lowe

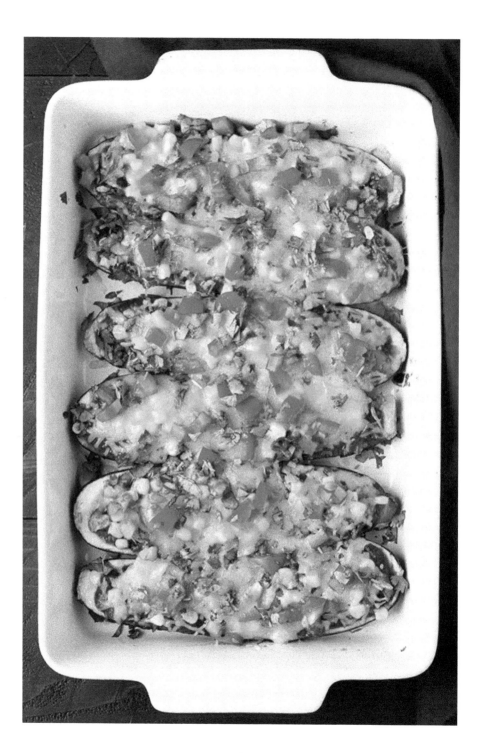

sources. Please consult a licensed professional before attempting any techniques outlined in this book.

By reading this document, the reader agrees that under no circumstances is the author responsible for any losses, direct or indirect, which are incurred as a result of the use of information contained within this document, including, but not limited to, — errors, omissions, or inaccuracies.

Table of Contents

French Onion Dip

Preparation time: 15 minutes

Cooking time: 9 hours

Servings: 8

Ingredients:

- 3 white onions, peeled and thinly sliced
- 1/2 teaspoon garlic powder
- 2 cups sour cream
- 1/2 cup mayonnaise
- 2 tablespoons melted coconut oil

Directions:

1. Add the onions and coconut oil to a 4-quarts slow-cooker. Cook within 7 to 9 hours. Allow cooking at a low heat setting, occasionally stirring until the onion has caramelized.

2. Leave the onion to cool until it reaches room temperature, then transfer them to a bowl and add the remaining ingredients. Flavor it with salt plus ground black pepper, mix all ingredients well. Serve as a dip with vegetables.

Nutrition:

- Calories: 522
- Carbohydrates: 12.8g
- Fats: 51.7g
- Protein: 3.5g

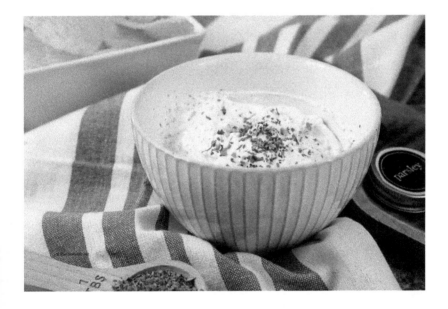

Queso Dip

Preparation time: 15 minutes

Cooking time: 2 hours & 30 minutes

Servings: 8

Ingredients:

- 8oz. cream cheese, cubed
- 8oz. Monterey Jack cheese
- 12oz. Salsa Verde

Directions:

1. Place all of the fixings in a 4-quart slow-cooker and stir until mixed. Cook within 2 1/2 hours. Allow cooking at a low heat setting, stirring every half hour. Puree the mixture with a stick blender, allow to cool, and serve with chopped vegetables.

Nutrition:

Calories: 171

Carbohydrates: 3g

Fats: 14g

Protein: 6g

Cauliflower Hummus

Preparation time: 15 minutes

Cooking time: 4 hours

Servings: 8

Ingredients:

- 3 cups cauliflower florets
- 5 garlic cloves, peeled
- 1 1/2 tablespoons tahini paste
- 2 tablespoons olive oil
- 3 tablespoons lemon juice

Directions:

1. Place the cauliflower florets in a 4-quart slow-cooker, add 3 garlic cloves and 1/4 cup water, and season with a pinch of salt.

2. Cover and seal the slow-cooker with its lid, and adjust the cooking timer for 3 to 4 hours. Allow cooking at a low heat setting.

3. Pulse the cauliflower mixture with a stick blender until smooth. Add the remaining ingredients and pulse again

with a stick blender until smooth. Adjust the seasoning, drizzle with olive oil and serve with chopped vegetables.

Nutrition:

- Calories: 141
- Carbohydrates: 7g
- Fats: 14g
- Protein: 2g

'Powerful 4' Chicken Wings

Preparation time: 15 minutes

Cooking time: 4 hours

Servings: 6

Ingredients:

- 6 chicken fillets
- 1 bottle hot sauce
- 4 tbsp butter, melted
- ½ packet ranch seasoning

Directions:

1. Make a mixture of hot sauce plus ranch seasoning, then coat the chicken pieces with it. Dissolve the butter in the slow-cooker, then put the chicken pieces at the bottom.

2. Cook without the lid for the first 30 minutes and then cook with the cover on a low setting for 3 hours 30 minutes. Serve with some of your favorite vegetables and sauce.

Nutrition:

- Calories: 140
- Carbs: 0g
- Fat: 18g
- Protein: 21g

Lamb Fillet

Preparation time: 15 minutes

Cooking time: 5 hours

Servings: 6

Ingredients:

- 6 lamb fillets, cut into ½ inch thick pieces
- 1 bottle hot sauce
- ½ cup tomato ketchup
- 4 tbsp butter, melted
- ½ packet ranch seasoning

Directions:

1. Make a mixture of hot sauce plus ranch seasoning and thoroughly coat the chicken pieces with it. Dissolve the butter in the slow cooker and place the chicken pieces at the bottom.

2. Cook without the lid within 30 minutes and then cook with the cover on low within 4 hours 30 minutes. Serve with some of your favorite vegetables and sauce.

Nutrition:

- Calories: 135
- Carbs: 0g
- Fat: 7g
- Protein: 27g

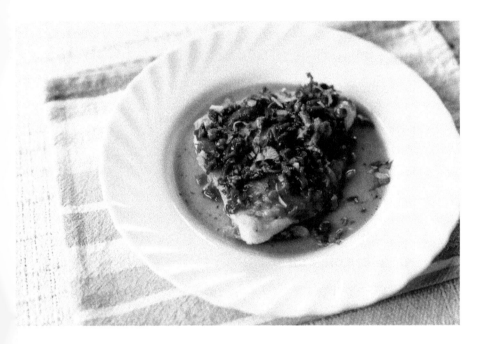

Chicken Rolls with Bean Sprouts

Preparation time: 15 minutes

Cooking time: 4 hours

Servings: 4

Ingredients:

- 4lb. chicken breast fillets
- 1 bunch asparagus, finely chopped
- 2 cloves of minced garlic
- 1 cup green beans sprout
- 1 cup grated mozzarella cheese
- 1 tsp salt
- 3 tbsp olive oil
- 1 tsp pepper

Directions:

1. Flatten the chicken fillets on the table using a wooden hammer. Put the green bean sprouts, garlic, salt, pepper, asparagus, plus grated cheese in a bowl and blend them properly.

2. Split the batter equally in 4 chicken fillets and cover the chicken tightly and secure with wooden toothpicks.

3. Put the chicken rolls in the slow cooker and cook on the low setting within 4 hours. Serve hot with your favorite sauce.

Nutrition:

- Calories: 150
- Carbs: 14g
- Fat: 7g
- Protein: 8g

Chicken & Mushroom Duet Roll

Preparation time: 15 minutes

Cooking time: 4 hours

Servings: 4

Ingredients:

- 4lb. chicken breast fillets
- 1 bunch asparagus, finely chopped
- 2 minced garlic cloves
- 1 cup chopped button mushrooms
- 1 cup grated mozzarella cheese
- 1 tsp salt
- 3 tbsp olive oil
- 1 tsp pepper

Directions:

1. Place the chicken fillets on the table and beat with a wooden hammer to flatten them. Cook the mushrooms in butter till they become slightly tender and light brown.

2. Now, put the cooked mushrooms, garlic, salt, pepper, asparagus, and grated cheese in a mixing bowl and blend them properly.

3. Divide the mixture equally into 4 chicken fillets and wrap the chicken tightly and secure with wooden toothpicks.

4. Put the chicken rolls in the slow cooker and cook with the lid on a low setting for 4 hours. Serve hot with your favorite sauce.

Nutrition:
- Calories: 618
- Carbs: 60g
- Fat: 18g
- Protein: 54g

Chicken Wings with the Bliss of Almond Butter

Preparation time: 15 minutes

Cooking time: 2 hours & 30 minutes

Servings : 4

Ingredients:

- 3 lb. chicken wings, half-cooked
- 4oz. almond butter
- ¾ cup hot sauce

Directions:

1. Heat the almond butter in the slow-cooker, and as soon as it melts, put in the semi-cooked chicken wings along with the hot sauce.

2. Blend them thoroughly and then cook without covering the cooker for 30 minutes. Now, cover the cooker and cook within 2 hours on a low setting. Serve hot with ketogenic buns.

Nutrition:

- Calories: 240
- Carbs: 13g
- Fat: 15g
- Protein: 15g

Chicken Drumsticks with Exotic Maple Flavor

Preparation time: 15 minutes

Cooking time: 2 hours & 30 minutes

Servings: 4

Ingredients:

- 4lb. chicken drumsticks (cooked till they are brown)
- 1 tsp ground cumin
- ½ cup lemon juice
- 1 tsp black pepper
- 1 tsp cayenne powder
- 1 tsp chili powder
- 1 tsp salt
- 4 tbsp unsweetened Maple Syrup
- 2 tbsp chopped cilantro
- 2 tbsp olive oil

Directions:

1. Put all the fixing in a mixing bowl, blend them well, and allow some time for marinating. Now heat olive oil in the slow-cooker and put the marinated chicken into it.

2. Cook without the cover for the first 30 minutes and remember to stir frequently. Now, put on the lid and cook on low setting for 2 hours. Make sure that the chicken is tender. Serve hot.

Nutrition:

- Calories: 140
- Carbs: 2g
- Fat: 6g
- Protein: 19g

Broccoli Magic with Twist of Ginger

Preparation time: 15 minutes

Cooking time: 3 hours & 30 minutes

Servings: 4

Ingredients:

- 1 large broccoli, cut into small florets
- 1 tsp ground black pepper
- 2 tbsp chopped cilantro
- 2 tbsp olive oil
- 1 tsp chili powder
- 1 tsp ground cumin
- 1 tsp salt
- 1 tsp cayenne pepper
- ½ cup lemon juice
- 2½ tsp minced ginger

Directions:

1. Put the broccoli florets in a bowl and add cilantro, lemon juice, black pepper, cayenne pepper, chili powder, cumin, and minced ginger.

2. Heat olive oil in the slow-cooker and put the broccoli mixture into it. Stir with a spatula and cook without cover for the first 30 minutes. Now cover the cooker and cook for 4 hours on a low setting. Serve warm.

Nutrition:

- Calories: 290
- Carbs: 17g
- Fat: 12g
- Protein: 27g

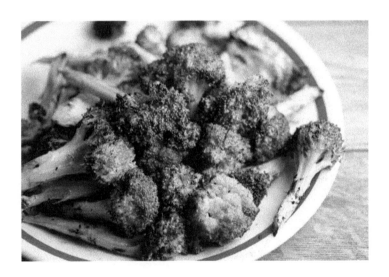

Super Cheesy Vegetable Roll

Preparation time: 15 minutes

Cooking time: 4 hours

Servings: 4

Ingredients:

- 4 large lettuce leaves
- ½ cup spinach puree
- 1 cup mozzarella cheese, grated
- ½ cup grated parmesan cheese
- 1 cup green beans sprout
- 2 garlic cloves, minced
- 1 bunch asparagus, finely chopped
- 3 tbsp olive oil
- Salt and pepper, according to taste

Directions:

1. Put bean sprouts, asparagus, garlic, spinach puree, salt, pepper, and grated cheese in a bowl and mix them well.

2. Divide this mixture equally over the lettuce leaves and wrap them tightly. Use fine threads to secure the wrapping.

3. Place the lettuce wraps at the bottom of a slow-cooker and pour olive oil from the top. Cover the cooker and cook on low setting for 4 hours. Remove the threads and serve hot with sauce.

Nutrition:

- Calories: 206
- Carbs: 37g
- Fat: 4g
- Protein: 5g

Healthy Spinach Magic Peppers

Preparation time: 15 minutes

Cooking time: 2 hours

Servings: 4

Ingredients:

- 4 large green bell peppers
- 2 lb. frozen spinach
- 2 tsp dried oregano
- 2 cups tomato paste
- 1 medium onion, diced
- 2 tsp thyme
- Salt and pepper, according to taste
- 2 tbsp basil, minced
- 3 garlic cloves, minced
- 2 tbsp olive oil
- 4 tbsp melted butter
- ½ cup mozzarella cheese

Directions:

1. Put olive oil in the slow-cooker and sauté onion and garlic till they become fragrant. Now add the spinach and cook till the leaves wilt completely.

2. Add basil, tomato paste, oregano, thyme, salt, and pepper and cook them for 20 minutes without the lid. By this time, the spinach leaves will form a smooth mixture. Transfer the mixture into a bowl and let it cool down completely.

3. Add the cheese to this mixture to prepare the stuffing for bell peppers. Put the stuffing into the bell pepper shells and coat them with the melted butter.

4. Keep the stuffed bell peppers at the bottom of the slow-cooker and pour the remaining butter from the top. Cook on the low setting within 2 hours and then serve.

Nutrition:

- Calories: 224
- Carbs: 12g
- Fat: 12g
- Protein: 19g

Keto-Fied Apple Cider

Preparation time : 15 minutes

Cooking time: 3 hours

Servings: 15

Ingredients:

- ¼ cup of coconut sugar
- ¼ cup of maple syrup
- 1 sliced navel orange
- 1 tsp. allspice berries
- 2 tsp. whole cloves
- 3 cinnamon sticks
- 6 apples of choice, cored and sliced
- 7 cups of water

Directions:

1. Pour all the fixing into your slow cooker and pour water over everything. Set to cook on high for 3 hours. Discard orange slices and cinnamon sticks.

2. Blend mixture using an immersion blender. Cook for another hour on high. Strain mixture through cheesecloth. Put it back in the pot to keep warm. Serve.

Nutrition:

- Calories: 178
- Carbs: 1g
- Fat: 8g
- Protein: 5g

Chocolate Chip Blueberry Cake

Preparation time: 15 minutes

Cooking time: 3 hours

Servings: 12

Ingredients:

- ¼ cup of chocolate whey protein powder
- ¼ cup of melted butter
- ¼ cup of melted coconut oil
- ¼ tsp. salt
- ½ cup of heavy cream
- ½ swerve sweetener
- 1 cup of blackberries
- 1 cup of unsweetened shredded coconut
- 1/3 cup dark chocolate chips (sugar-free)
- 2 cups of almond flour
- 2 tsp. baking soda
- 4 eggs

Directions:

1. Grease inside of a slow cooker with butter. Mix all of the dry ingredients. Then add in all wet components, blending well to ensure adequate incorporation.

2. Pour batter into the prepared slow cooker. Set to cook on low 3 hours. Top with additional blueberries before indulging.

Nutrition:

- Calories: 289
- Carbs: 5g
- Fat: 19g
- Protein: 9g

Zesty Lemon Cake

Preparation time: 15 minutes

Cooking time: 8 hours

Servings: 10

Ingredients:

- ¼ cup of coconut flour
- ¼ cup of plain egg protein powder
- ½ cup of unsweetened almond milk
- ½ cup of swerve sweetener
- 1 tsp. baking soda
- 1/3 cup of butter
- 2 cups of almond flour
- 2 tsp. cream of tartar
- 2 tsp. vanilla extract
- 4 eggs
- Zest of 1 lemon

Filling:

- 1 cup of coconut cream
- 1 cup of low-carb lemon curd
- 1 tsp. vanilla extract

Glaze:

- ½ cup of coconut butter
- 1 tbsp. lemon juice
- 2 tbsp. coconut oil
- 2 tbsp. swerve sweetener
- Zest of 1 lemon

Directions:

1. Combine almond milk and butter. Then mix in vanilla, eggs, and lemon zest. Combine all dry components. Then combine wet and dry mixtures, blending well.

2. Line a springform pan with parchment paper and pour batter into it. Place pan into the slow cooker and cook on low 2 hours. Take out and place in the fridge 4-6 hour to chill.

3. For the filling, combine all ingredients until smooth. Do the same with glaze. Cut cake in half. Fill one part of the cake with a filling, lay the other half over the top, and then drizzle with glaze. Tip with additional lemon zest.

Nutrition:

- Calories: 250
- Carbs: 2g
- Fat: 16g
- Protein: 11g

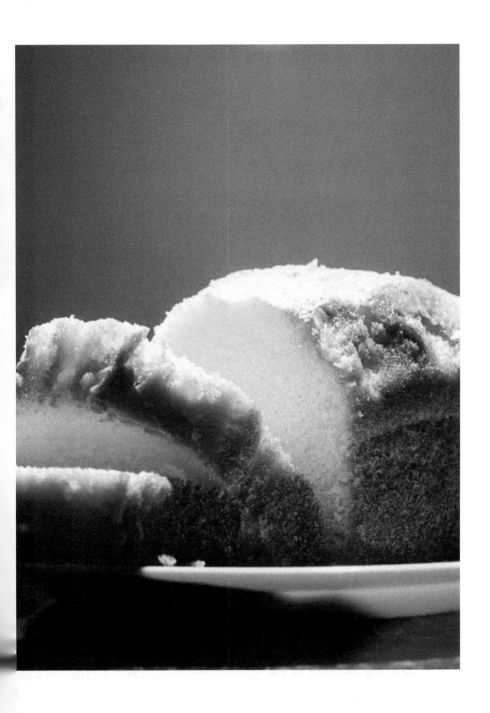

Keto Cheesecake

Preparation time: 15 minutes

Cooking time: 3 hours

Servings: 12

Ingredients:

- ½ tbsp. vanilla extract
- 1 cup of Splenda
- 3 8-ounce packages of cream cheese
- 3 eggs

Directions:

1. Let the cream cheese to warm up at room temperature. Mix sugar and cream cheese until well blended. Mix in one egg at a time, making sure to beat well after every addition.

2. Add vanilla and mix well. Grease a pan or bowl well and add cream cheese mixture to it. Add 2-3 cups of water into the bottom of the slow cooker. Add pan to pot. Set to cook on high 2 – 2 ½ hours.

Nutrition:

- Calories: 301
- Carbs: 2g
- Fat: 31g
- Protein: 23g

Creamy Pumpkin Custard

Preparation time: 15 minutes

Cooking time: 3 hours

Servings: 10

Ingredients:

- 4 tbsp. butter
- 1 tsp. pumpkin pie spice
- ½ cup of almond flour
- 1 tsp. vanilla extract
- 1 cup of pumpkin puree
- ½ cup of granulated stevia
- 4 eggs
- 1/8 tsp. Salt

Directions:

1. Grease inside of a slow cooker. Beat eggs until smooth. Then beat in sweetener gradually. Add vanilla and pumpkin puree until blended well.

2. Then mix in pumpkin pie spice, salt, and almond flour. Blend as you add in butter. Pour into a slow cooker.

3. Place a paper towel over the opening of the pot before closing it. Cook 2-3 hours on low. Serve warm with whipped cream and a dash of nutmeg!

Nutrition:

- Calories: 419
- Carbs: 4g
- Fat: 16g
- Protein: 19g

Chocolate Molten Lava Cake

Preparation time: 15 minutes

Cooking time: 3 hours

Servings: 12

Ingredients:

- ½ cup of melted and cooled butter
- ½ cup of flour
- ½ tsp. salt
- ½ tsp. vanilla liquid stevia
- 1 ½ cup of swerve sweetener
- 1 tsp. baking powder
- 1 tsp. vanilla extract
- 2 cups of hot water
- 3 egg yolks
- 3 whole eggs
- 4-ounces sugar-free chocolate chips
- 5 tbsp. unsweetened cocoa powder

Directions:

1. Grease slow cooker liberally. Whisk baking powder, salt, 3 tbsp cocoa powder, flour, and 1 ¼ cup of swerve sweetener. Stir liquid stevia, vanilla, yolks, eggs, and melted butter.

2. Combine wet and dry mixture till well incorporated. Pour into a slow cooker. Top with chocolate chips. Mix in the remaining swerve and cocoa powder. Set to cook on low 3 hours.

Nutrition:

- Calories: 418
- Carbs: 4g
- Fat: 27g
- Protein: 8g

Lemon Slow Cooker Cake

Preparation time: 15 minutes

Cooking time: 3 hours

Servings: 8

Ingredients:

- ½ cup of coconut flour
- ½ cup of melted butter
- ½ cup of whipping cream
- ½ tsp. xanthan gum
- 1 ½ cup of almond flour
- 2 eggs
- 2 tbsp. lemon juice
- 2 tsp. baking powder
- 3 tbsp. swerve sweetener
- Zest of 2 lemons

Topping:

- ½ cup of boiling water
- 2 tbsp. lemon juice
- 2 tbsp. melted butter
- 3 tbsp. swerve sweetener

Directions:

1. Combine xanthan gum, baking powder, sweetener, and flours. Whisk egg, lemon juice and zest, whipping cream, and butter.

2. Mix dry and wet components and pour the mixture into your greased slow cooker.

3. For the topping, combine all topping components till incorporated and spread over top of cake mixture. Set to cook on high 2-3 hours. Serve warm with whipped cream and fresh fruit!

Nutrition:

- Calories: 310
- Carbs: 4g
- Fat: 29g
- Protein: 8g

Keto Chocolate Cake

Preparation time: 15 minutes

Cooking time: 2 hours & 30 minutes

Servings: 7

Ingredients:

- ¼ tsp. salt
- ½ cup of cocoa powder
- ½ cup of Swerve sweetener
- ¾ tsp. vanilla extract
- 1 ½ tsp. baking powder
- 1 cup + 2 tbsp. almond flour
- 1/3 cup of sugar-free chocolate chips
- 2/3 cup of unsweetened almond milk
- 3 eggs
- 3 tbsp. whey protein powder
- 6 tbsp. melted butter

Directions:

1. Grease slow cooker. Mix salt, baking powder, protein powder, cocoa powder, sweetener, and almond flour.

2. Mix in vanilla, almond milk, eggs, and butter. Fold in chocolate chips. Pour into a slow cooker. Set to cook on low 2 ½ hours. Let cool and then slice into pieces.

Nutrition:
- Calories: 357
- Carbs: 5g
- Fat: 26g
- Protein: 13g

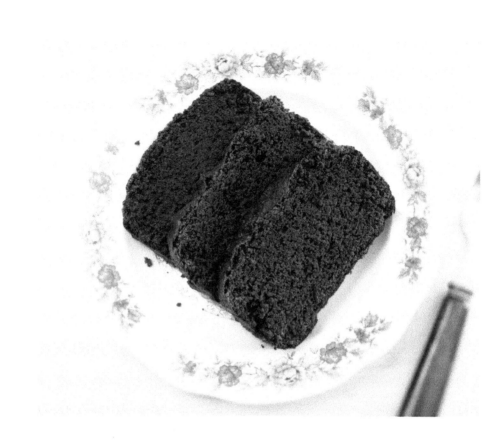

Blueberry Lemon Custard Cake

Preparation time: 15 minutes

Cooking time: 3 hours

Servings: 9

Ingredients:

- ½ cup of sweetener of choice
- ½ cup of coconut flour
- ½ cup of fresh blueberries
- ½ tsp. salt
- 1 tsp. lemon stevia
- 1/3 cup of lemon juice
- 2 cups of light cream
- 2 tsp. lemon zest
- 6 separated eggs

Directions:

1. Add egg whites to a stand mixer, whipping till soft peaks are made. Whisk yolks with remaining ingredients minus blueberries. Fold in egg whites.

2. Grease slow cooker and pour in batter. Sprinkle with blueberries. Set to cook on low 3 hours. Allow to cook at least 1 hour and then chill at least 2 hours or overnight. Serve ice cold with sugar-free whipped cream!

Nutrition:

- Calories: 375
- Carbs: 4g
- Fat: 27g
- Protein: 14g

Almond Carrot Cake

Preparation time: 15 minutes

Cooking time: 2 hours

Servings: 8

Ingredients:

- ¼ cup of coconut oil
- ½ cup of heavy whipping cream
- ½ cup of slivered almonds
- 1 ½ tsp. apple pie spice
- 1 cup of almond flour
- 1 cup of shredded carrots
- 1 tsp. baking powder
- 3 eggs

Directions:

1. Oiled a cake pan that will fit into the slow cooker. Mix all recipe components with an electric hand mixer, beating till fluffy and incorporated.

2. Pour batter into the pan, then cover it with foil. Pour 2 cups water into the bottom of the slow cooker. Place a

trivet over water and carefully place the pan onto the trivet.

3.   Cook cake for 2 hours on medium heat until done. Take out of the slow cooker and let cool before cutting and frosting to eat.

Nutrition:

- Calories: 268
- Carbs: 6g
- Fat: 21g
- Protein: 6g

Decadent Chocolate Cake

Preparation time: 15 minutes

Cooking time: 2 hours & 30 minutes

Servings: 6

Ingredients:

- ½ cup of unsalted butter
- ½ tsp. baking powder
- ¾ cup of almond flour
- ¾ cup of cocoa powder
- 1 ½ cup of powdered sweetener
- 1 tsp. vanilla extract
- 3 separated eggs

Directions:

1. Separate eggs. Beat whites with an electric mixer until fluffy. Put to the side. Then beat yolks till smooth and put to the side.

2. Combine baking powder, cocoa powder, and flour. Beat butter and powdered sweetener in a separate bowl until creamy.

3. Add egg whites to the butter mixture. Then beat in egg yolks with a hand mixer. Add vanilla and incorporate it well. Slowly pour in almond flour mixture to egg mixture, folding well after each new addition.

4. With parchment paper, line a cake pan. Grease with butter. Pour batter into prepared pan. Gently place the pan into the slow cooker and cook 2 ½ hours till done in the middle. Indulge without the guilt!

Nutrition:

- Calories: 312
- Carbs: 3g
- Fat: 18g
- Protein: 5g

Pumpkin Pie Pudding

Preparation time: 15 minutes

Cooking time: 3 hours

Servings: 6

Ingredients:

- ½ cup of heavy whipping cream
- ½ cup of heavy whipping cream (for finishing)
- ¾ cup of erythritol
- 1 tsp. pumpkin pie spice
- 1 tsp. vanilla extract
- 15 ounces canned pumpkin puree
- 2 eggs

Directions:

1. Whisk vanilla extract, pumpkin pie spice, pumpkin puree, erythritol, heavy whipping cream, and eggs. Grease a pan with butter (ensure you get in the corners well!)

2. Pour 1 ½ cups water into your slow cooker. Place a trivet over water. Pour batter into the pan and gently place the pan in a pressure cooker. Cover with a piece of foil.

3. Cook 2 ½ to 3 hours till well combined and custard-like. Before enjoying, chill 6-8 hours.

Nutrition:

- Calories: 184
- Carbs: 6g
- Fat: 16g
- Protein: 3g

Banana Nut Bread

Preparation time: 15 minutes

Cooking time: 2 hours

Servings: 6

Ingredients:

- ¼ cup of chopped nuts of choice
- ¼ cup of sweetener of choice
- ½ tsp. salt
- 1 ½ tsp. baking soda
- 1/3 cup of unsweetened applesauce
- 2 cup of low-carb baking mix
- 2 eggs
- 2 tbsp. room temp butter
- 2-3 ripe bananas

Directions:

1. Combine eggs, applesauce, butter, and sweetener. Beat with a hand mixer till smooth. Mash bananas and mix in. Add all dry components, incorporating well. Fold in nuts.

2. Oiled a pan and pour batter into it. Use a piece of foil to cover. Pour 1 cup of water into the slow cooker, then place a trivet over water and gently place the pan onto the trivet.

3. Cook 2 hours till bread is done in the middle. Let cool to room temp before eating.

Nutrition:

- Calories: 182
- Carbs: 8g
- Fat: 19g
- Protein: 11g

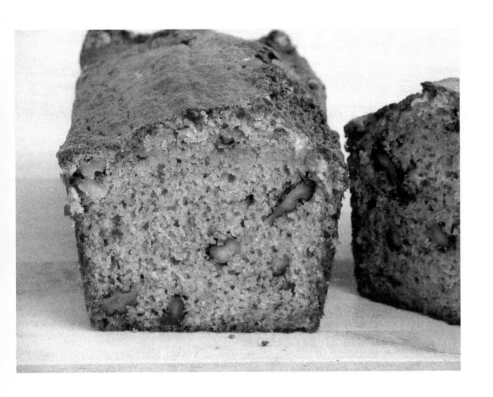

Sweet & Tangy Beef Shoulder

Preparation Time: 15 minutes

Cooking Time: 9 hours 10 minutes

Servings: 14

Ingredients:

- ¼ cup unsalted butter
- 8 pounds grass-fed chuck shoulder roast
- Salt
- Ground black pepper
- 1 yellow onion, chopped
- 4 garlic cloves, minced
- 1 tablespoon Dijon mustard
- 2 tablespoons vinegar
- 2 tablespoons fresh lemon juice
- 3-4 drops liquid stevia

Directions:

1. Dissolve the butter in a large skillet over medium-high heat and cook beef with salt and black pepper for about 1-2 minutes per side.

2. Transfer the beef into a large crockpot. In the same skillet, add onion and sauté for about 2-3 minutes. Place onion evenly over beef.

3. In a bowl, mix the remaining ingredients. Pour the sauce evenly over beef. Set the crockpot on low and cook, covered, for about 9 hours.

4. Uncover the crockpot and transfer the beef to a cutting board. Transfer the sauce into a small pan over medium-high heat and cook for about 5 minutes or until desired thickness.

5. Cut beef shoulder into desired sized slices. Pour sauce over beef slices and serve.

Nutrition:

- Calories: 516
- Carbohydrates: 1.1g
- Protein: 48.4g
- Fat: 33.1g

Succulent Beef Pot Roast

Preparation Time : 15 minutes

Cooking Time: 8 hours

Servings: 6

Ingredients:

- 2 pounds grass-fed beef pot roast
- 1 yellow onion, sliced
- 2 garlic cloves, minced
- 2 jalapeño peppers, minced
- 1 tablespoon fresh rosemary, minced
- ¼ cup fresh lemon juice
- ½ cup homemade beef broth
- 1 teaspoon ground cumin
- Salt
- Ground black pepper

Directions:

1. Put grass-fed beef pot roast, and other fixing in a large crockpot and stir to combine. Cook on low within 6-8 hours.

2. Uncover the crockpot and transfer the beef roast to a cutting board. Cut beef roast into desired sized slices and serve.

Nutrition:

- Calories: 298
- Carbohydrates: 2.6g
- Protein: 46.7g
- Fat: 9.9g

Divine Beef Shanks

Preparation Time: 15 minutes

Cooking Time: 8 hours 10 minutes

Servings: 10

Ingredients:

- 3 tablespoons unsalted butter
- 5 (1-pound) grass-fed beef shanks
- Salt
- Ground black pepper
- 1 large yellow onion, chopped
- 10 garlic cloves, minced
- 2 tablespoons sugar-free tomato paste
- 4 fresh rosemary sprigs
- 4 fresh thyme sprigs
- 2 cups homemade beef broth

Directions:

1. Dissolve the butter over medium-high heat in a large skillet and cook beef shanks with salt and black pepper for about 4-5 minutes per side.

2. Transfer the beef shanks to a large crockpot. In the same skillet, sauté onion for about 3-4 minutes. Add garlic and sauté within 1 minute.

3. Place onion mixture over beef shanks and cover evenly with tomato paste. With a kitchen string, tie the herbs sprigs.

4. Arrange tied sprigs over tomato paste and pour the broth on top evenly. Set the crockpot on low and cook, covered, for about 8 hours. Serve hot.

Nutrition:

- Calories: 513
- Carbohydrates: 3.2g
- Protein: 77.9g
- Fat: 18.9g

Family Dinner Beef Brisket

Preparation Time: 15 minutes

Cooking Time: 6 hours

Servings: 12

Ingredients:

- 1 large yellow onion, sliced
- 3 garlic cloves, chopped
- 1 (4-pound) grass-fed beef brisket
- ½ teaspoon red pepper flakes, crushed
- ½ teaspoon smoked paprika
- ½ teaspoon ground cumin
- Salt
- Ground black pepper
- 2 cups homemade beef broth

Directions:

1. In a large crockpot, put all the fixing and stir to combine. Cook on low, covered, within 6 hours. Uncover the crockpot and transfer the beef brisket onto a cutting board. Cut beef brisket into desired sized slices and serve.

Nutrition:

- Calories: 353

- Carbohydrates: 2g
- Protein: 56.3g
- Fat: 11.6g

Italian Beef Stroganoff

Preparation Time: 15 minutes

Cooking Time: 8 hours

Servings: 8

Ingredients:

- 4 pounds grass-fed beef short ribs
- ½ teaspoon red pepper flakes, crushed
- Salt
- Ground black pepper
- 1 cup button mushrooms, sliced
- 1½ cups tomatoes, chopped finely
- ½ cup onion, chopped
- 4 garlic cloves, minced
- 2 tablespoons fresh basil leaves, chopped
- 2 cups homemade beef broth
- ½ cup dry white wine

Directions:

1. In a large crockpot, put all the listed fixing, then stir. Set the crockpot on low and cook, covered, for about 4-6 hours. Serve hot.

Nutrition:

- Calories: 500
- Carbohydrates: 3.5g
- Protein: 67.5g
- Fat: 20.9g

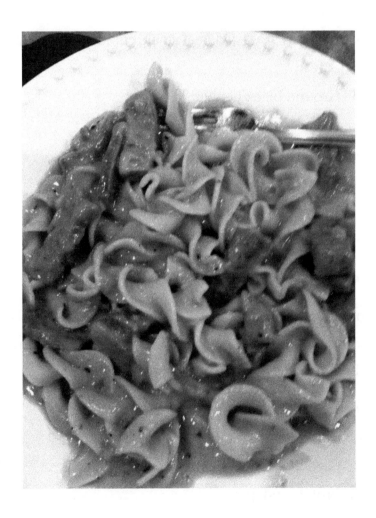

Energizing Beef Casserole

Preparation Time: 20 minutes

Cooking Time: 9 hours

Servings: 5

Ingredients:

- 1-pound grass-fed beef steak, cut into thin strips
- Salt
- Ground black pepper
- 1 small yellow onion, sliced
- 1 cup tomatoes, chopped
- 1 cup fresh mushrooms, sliced
- 1¼ cups fresh green beans
- ½ cup homemade beef broth

Directions:

1. In a large crockpot, put all the above fixing and stir to combine. Set the crockpot on low and cook, covered, for about 8 hours. Serve hot.

Nutrition:

- Calories: 196
- Carbohydrates: 5.2g
- Protein: 29.4g

- Fat: 5.9g

North American Pork Ribs

Preparation Time: 20 minutes

Cooking Time: 10 hours

Servings: 6

Ingredients:

- 3 pounds pork ribs
- 1 small yellow onion, chopped
- 2 garlic cloves, minced
- 1 cup baby carrots, peeled and chopped
- ½ cup homemade chicken broth
- ¼ cup coconut aminos
- 1 tablespoon olive oil
- Salt
- Ground black pepper

Directions:

1. In a large crockpot, add all ingredients and stir to combine. Set the crockpot on low and cook, covered, within 8-10 hours. Serve hot.

Nutrition:

- Calories: 506
- Carbohydrates: 5.8g

- Protein: 45.9g
- Fat: 32g

Simply Delicious Pork Chops

Preparation Time: 15 minutes

Cooking Time: 5 hours 5 minutes

Servings: 5

Ingredients:

- 1 tablespoon coconut oil
- 2 garlic cloves, minced
- 5 (4-ounce) boneless pork chops
- Salt
- Ground black pepper
- 1 large zucchini, cubed
- 2 lemons, sliced
- 1 teaspoon red pepper flakes, crushed

Directions:

1. In a large skillet, heat-up oil on medium-high heat and sauté garlic for about 1 minute. Add chops and cook for 1-2 minutes per side.

2. Transfer the chops mixture into a crockpot. Place cubed zucchini over chops evenly, followed by lemon slices.

3. Sprinkle with red pepper flakes, salt, and black pepper. Set the crockpot on High and cook, covered, for about 5 hours. Serve hot

Nutrition:

- Calories: 206
- Carbohydrates: 4.9g
- Protein: 30.8g
- Fat: 7g

Fall-of-the-Bone Pork Shoulder

Preparation Time: 15 minutes

Cooking Time: 8 hours 10 minutes

Servings: 8

Ingredients:

- 2 tablespoons olive oil
- 3 pounds of pork shoulder
- Salt
- Ground black pepper
- 1 medium yellow onion, chopped
- 1 celery stalk, chopped
- 2 garlic cloves, minced
- 2 cups fresh tomatoes, chopped finely
- ½ cup homemade chicken broth
- 2 tablespoons fresh lemon juice

Directions:

1. In a large skillet, heat-up oil on medium-high heat and cook pork shoulder with salt and black pepper for about 4-5 minutes per side.

2. Transfer pork shoulder to a crockpot and top with onion, celery, garlic, and tomatoes. Pour broth and lemon juice on top.

3. Set the crockpot on low and cook, covered, for about 8 hours. Uncover the crockpot and transfer the pork shoulder onto a cutting board. Cut pork shoulder into desired sized slices and serve.

Nutrition:

- Calories: 545
- Carbohydrates: 3.5g
- Protein: 40.5g
- Fat: 40.1g

Christmas Dinner Pork Roast

Preparation Time: 15 minutes

Cooking Time: 8 hours

Servings: 10

Ingredients:

- 4 pounds boneless pork roast
- 1 teaspoon dried rosemary, crushed
- 1 teaspoon dried thyme, crushed
- 1 teaspoon cayenne pepper
- ½ teaspoon smoked paprika
- Salt
- Ground black pepper
- 1 medium yellow onion, sliced thinly and divided
- 1 cup hot homemade chicken broth

Directions:

1. Rub the pork with herbs and spices generously. At the bottom of a large crockpot, place half the onion and top with pork roast, followed by the remaining onion.

2. Pour broth on top. Set the crockpot on low and cook, covered, for about 6-8 hours. Uncover the crockpot and

transfer the pork roast onto a cutting board. Cut pork roast into desired sized slices and serve.

Nutrition:

- Calories: 269
- Carbohydrates: 1.4g
- Protein: 48.1g
- Fat: 17.5g

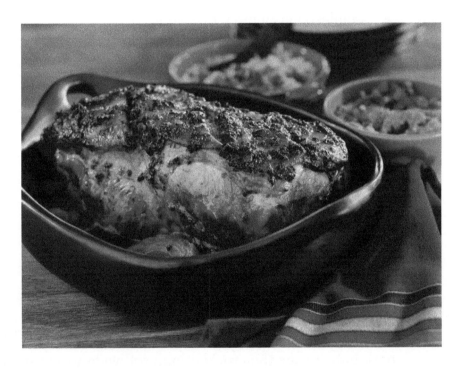

Asian Style Pork Butt

Preparation Time: 15 minutes

Cooking Time : 8 hours

Servings: 8

Ingredients:

- 1 medium onion, sliced thinly
- 4 garlic cloves, minced
- 3 tablespoons lemongrass, minced
- 1 tablespoon vinegar
- 3 tablespoons olive oil
- Salt
- Ground black pepper
- 3 pounds pork butt, trimmed
- 1 cup unsweetened coconut milk

Directions:

1. In a large bowl, add garlic, lemongrass, vinegar, oil, and seasoning. Rub the pork butt with garlic mixture evenly.

2. In a large crockpot, place the onion slices and top with pork butt. Cover the crockpot and set aside to marinate for at least 8 hours.

3. Uncover the crockpot and pour coconut milk on top. Set the crockpot on low and cook, covered, for about 8 hours.

4. Uncover the crockpot and transfer the pork butt onto a cutting board. Cut pork butt into desired sized slices and serve.

Nutrition:

- Calories: 445
- Carbohydrates: 3.9g
- Protein: 53.9g
- Fat: 23.8g

Meaty Pie

Preparation time: 15 minutes

Cooking time: 6 hours & 30 minutes

Servings: 6

Ingredients:

- 1 ½ pounds ground beef
- 1 egg
- ½ cup almonds ground finely into a flour
- ½ cup Parmesan cheese, freshly grated
- ½ cup green bell pepper, diced
- ½ cup onion, diced
- 1 teaspoon salt
- 1 teaspoon black pepper
- 1 tablespoon fresh oregano
- 2 cups tomatoes, chopped
- 2 garlic cloves, crushed and minced
- ½ cup fresh basil, chopped
- 1 cup fresh Mozzarella, sliced

Directions:

1. Mix the ground beef, egg, almonds, Parmesan cheese, green bell pepper, and onion in a bowl. Flavor the mixture with salt, black pepper, plus oregano. Mix well.

2. Take the meat mixture and press it firmly into the bottom of the slow cooker. Place the tomatoes, garlic, and basil in a blender and puree. Pour the tomato mixture over the meat. Cover and cook on low within 6 hours.

3. Remove the lid and arrange the mozzarella cheese slices over the top. Replace the cover and cook within 30 minutes before serving.

Nutrition:

- Calories: 406.7
- Fat: 31.7g
- Carbs: 7.2g
- Protein: 23.7g

Mexican Meatloaf

Preparation time: 15 minutes

Cooking time: 7 hours

Servings: 6

Ingredients:

- 1 ½ pounds ground beef
- 1 egg
- 1 cup añejo cheese, grated
- 1 cup onion, diced
- 2 tablespoons jalapeño pepper, diced
- ¼ cup fresh cilantro, chopped
- 2 teaspoons chili powder
- 1 teaspoon ground cumin
- 1 teaspoon salt
- 1 teaspoon black pepper
- 1 cup roasted tomatoes, chopped
- ½ cup Mexican crema
- 1 avocado, sliced

Directions:

1. Mix the ground beef, egg, añejo cheese, onion, and jalapeño pepper in a bowl. Season the mixture with the

cilantro, chili powder, cumin, salt, and black pepper. Mix well.

2. Line a slow cooker with aluminum foil for easier removal, if desired. Take the meat mixture and either form it into a loaf, place it in the slow cooker, or press the meat mixture into the slow cooker's bottom.

3. Add the tomatoes on top of the meatloaf. Cover and cook on low for 7 hours, or until cooked through. Serve garnished with a dollop of Mexican crema and sliced avocado.

Nutrition:

- Calories: 545.2
- Fat: 45.6g
- Carbs: 8.3g
- Protein: 26.7g

Whiskey Blues Steak

Preparation time: 15 minutes

Cooking time: 6 hours

Servings: 6

Ingredients:

- 1 ½ pound beef steak
- 1 teaspoon salt
- 2 teaspoons coarsely ground black pepper
- 3 cups zucchini, sliced thick
- ¼ cup butter
- 1 cup onions, sliced
- ¼ cup whiskey
- 2 garlic cloves, crushed and minced
- ½ cup blue cheese, crumbled

Directions:

1. Flavor the steak with salt plus black pepper. Place the sliced zucchini in the bottom of the slow cooker.

2. Melt the butter in a skillet over medium-high heat. Add the steaks to the skillet and brown on both sides, approximately 2-4 minutes.

3. Remove the steaks from the skillet and place them in the slow cooker. Add the onions to the skillet and sauté until crisp-tender, approximately 3-4 minutes.

4. Add the whiskey and cook until reduced, 1-2 minutes, scraping the bottom of the skillet. Put the onions back in the slow cooker and sprinkle in the garlic.

5. Cover and cook on low within 6 hours, or until the steaks are cooked to the desired doneness and are tender. Serve the steaks garnished with blue cheese.

Nutrition:

- Calories: 305
- Fat: 15.4g
- Carbs: 6.1g
- Protein: 29.2g

Philly Cheese Steak

Preparation time: 15 minutes

Cooking time: 4 hours & 30 minutes

Servings: 6

Ingredients:

- 1 cup green bell pepper, sliced
- 1 cup onion, sliced
- ¼ cup of butter melted
- 1 ½ pound beef steak, sliced thin
- 4 garlic cloves, crushed and minced
- ¼ cup Worcestershire sauce
- ¼ cup beef stock
- ¼ cup of soy sauce
- 1 teaspoon salt
- 1 teaspoon black pepper
- 1 teaspoon paprika
- 1 cup Swiss cheese, shredded
- Bibb lettuce leaves or approved keto bread for serving (optional)

Directions:

1. Place the green bell pepper and the onion in a slow cooker. Pour in the butter and toss to coat. Add the sliced beef steak into the slow cooker.

2. In a bowl, combine the garlic, Worcestershire sauce, beef stock, soy sauce, salt, black pepper, and paprika. Mix well and pour the liquid into the slow cooker.

3. Cook on high within 4 hours. Remove the lid and sprinkle in the Swiss cheese. Replace the cover, turn the heat to low, and cook an additional 30 minutes before serving.

Nutrition:

- Calories: 312.6
- Fat: 17.1g
- Carbs: 6.6g
- Protein: 32.2g

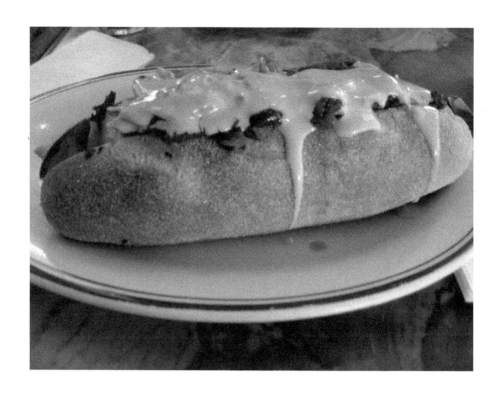

Steak Stuffed Peppers

Preparation time: 15 minutes

Cooking time : 4 hours

Servings: 4

Ingredients:

- 4 red bell peppers
- 2 tablespoons butter
- 1-pound beef steak, sliced thin
- 1 teaspoon salt
- 1 teaspoon black pepper
- 1 tablespoon fresh rosemary, finely chopped
- ¼ cup fresh basil, chopped
- 4 garlic cloves, crushed and minced
- 1 cup tomatoes, chopped
- ½ cup onion, diced
- ½ cup celery, diced
- ½ cup walnuts, chopped
- ½ cup Stilton cheese, crumbled
- 1 cup beef stock or water

Directions:

1. Slice the bell pepper's tops off and scoop the seeds out. Dissolve the butter over medium heat in a skillet. Place the steak in the skillet and cook for 1-2 minutes.

2. Season the steak with salt, black pepper, rosemary, basil, and garlic. Add the tomatoes and cook for an additional 2-3 minutes. Remove, then allow it to cool enough to handle.

3. Combine the steak with the onion, celery, walnuts, and Stilton cheese. Scoop equal amounts of the steak mixture into each of the peppers. Pour the beef stock or water into the slow cooker.

4. Replace the tops on the peppers and arrange them in the slow cooker. Cover and cook on high within 4 hours.

Nutrition:

- Calories: 397
- Fat: 26.4g
- Carbs: 11.0g
- Protein: 33.0g

Spicy Citrus Meatballs

Preparation time: 15 minutes

Cooking time: 8 hours

Servings: 6

Ingredients:

- 1 ½ pounds ground beef
- 1 egg
- 1 tablespoon Worcestershire sauce
- 1 tablespoon garlic chili sauce
- ½ cup onion, diced
- 1 cup zucchini, shredded
- 2 tablespoons olive oil
- 3 cups green beans, trimmed
- 1 cup beef stock
- 1 tablespoon crushed red pepper flakes
- ¼ cup of soy sauce
- 1 teaspoon orange extract
- 1 teaspoon black pepper

Directions:

1. Mix the ground beef, egg, Worcestershire sauce, garlic chili sauce, onion, and zucchini in a bowl. Take spoonsful

of the meat mixture and form them into golf ball-sized meatballs.

2.   Pour the olive oil into a skillet over medium heat. Place the meatballs in the skillet and cook just until browned on all sides. Place the green beans in the slow cooker.

3.   Transfer the meatballs from the skillet to the slow cooker. Combine the beef stock, crushed red pepper flakes, soy sauce, orange extract, and black pepper, then put into the slow cooker. Cover and cook on low within 8 hours.

Nutrition:

- Calories: 434.6
- Fat: 35.8g
- Carbs: 6.5g
- Protein: 21.7g

Swedish Broccoli and Meatballs

Preparation time: 15 minutes

Cooking time: 7 hours & 30 minutes

Servings: 6

Ingredients:

- 1-pound ground beef
- ½ cup onion, diced
- ½ cup celery, diced
- 2 garlic cloves, crushed and minced
- 1 cup heavy cream, divided
- ½ cup Parmesan cheese, freshly grated
- 1 tablespoon olive oil
- 4 cups broccoli florets
- 1 teaspoon salt
- 1 teaspoon black pepper
- ¼ cup butter, melted
- ½ cup sour cream
- 1 tablespoon fresh chives
- 1 tablespoon fresh thyme

Directions:

1.   Mix the ground beef, onion, celery, garlic, ¼ cup of the heavy cream, and the Parmesan cheese in a bowl.

2.   Get a spoonful of it, then form them into meatballs measuring approximately one inch in diameter. Heat-up olive oil in a skillet over medium heat.

3.   Place the meatballs in the skillet and cook just until browned. Place the broccoli, seasoned with salt and black pepper, in the slow cooker, followed by the butter. Toss to coat.

4.   Transfer the meatballs from the skillet to the slow cooker. Cover and cook on low for 7 hours. Combine the remaining heavy cream, sour cream, chives, and thyme.

5.   Lift the lid off the slow cooker, add the cream mixture, and stir. Replace the lid and cook an additional 30 minutes before serving.

Nutrition:

- Calories: 561.2
- Fat: 51.4g
- Carbs: 6.8g
- Protein: 19.5g

Balsamic Dijon Short Ribs

Preparation time: 15 minutes

Cooking time: 8 hours

Servings: 6

Ingredients:

- 2 pounds beef short ribs
- 1 teaspoon salt
- 1 teaspoon black pepper
- 2 tablespoons olive oil
- 2 cups Napa cabbage, shredded
- ¼ cup balsamic vinegar
- ¼ cup Dijon mustard
- ½ cup beef stock
- 1 tablespoon fresh thyme
- 2 garlic cloves, crushed and minced

Directions:

1. Flavor the ribs with salt plus black pepper. Heat-up olive oil in a skillet over medium heat. Place the ribs in the skillet and cook for 1-2 minutes per side.

2. Spread the cabbage in the bottom of the slow cooker. Transfer the ribs from the skillet to the slow cooker.

3. Combine the balsamic vinegar, Dijon mustard, beef stock, thyme, garlic, and mix well. Pour the mixture over the ribs. Cover and cook on low within 8 hours.

Nutrition:

- Calories: 282.1
- Fat: 15.4g
- Carbs: 1.8g
- Protein: 30.4g

Slow Cooker Winter Veggies

Preparation time: 15 minutes

Cooking time: 3 hours

Servings: 4

Ingredients:

- 2 cups sliced leeks
- 1 cup carrots, sliced
- 1 ½ cups red onion, diced
- 2 cups butternut squash, diced
- 1 cup celery, sliced
- ½ cup of balsamic vinegar
- ½ cup olive oil
- 2 tablespoons fresh mint, chopped
- 1 tablespoon fresh dill, chopped

Directions:

1. Combine the vegetables in a large bowl. Combine the olive oil and balsamic in another bowl. Stir in the mint and dill.

2. Place vegetables in your slow cooker and cover with the marinade. Stir until the vegetables are cooked entirely. Cook on high for three hours, stirring every hour.

Nutrition:

- Calories: 233
- Fat: 18g
- Protein: 3g
- Carbs: 18g

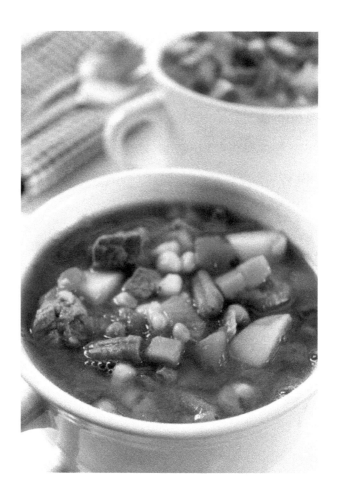

Cauliflower Breakfast Casserole

Preparation time: 15 minutes

Cooking time: 5 hours

Servings: 4

Ingredients:

- 1 egg
- ½ cup milk
- ½ teaspoon dry mustard
- 1 teaspoon salt
- ½ teaspoon pepper
- 1 head cauliflower, shredded
- 1 onion, diced
- 2 5-ounce packages vegetarian sausage crumbles
- 2 cups of shredded cheddar cheese

Directions:

1. Beat the eggs, milk, dry mustard, and salt and pepper. Place one-third of the shredded cauliflower at the bottom of the slow cooker, then add one-third of the onion. Sprinkle with salt and pepper.

2. Add one-third of the vegetarian sausage and cheddar cheese. Repeat these two more times. Pour the egg

mixture over everything, cover, and cook on low for 5 hours or until the top is browned.

Nutrition:

- Calories: 215
- Fat: 18g
- Protein: 3g
- Carbs: 18g

Mexican Cauliflower Rice

Preparation time: 15 minutes

Cooking time: 4 hours

Servings: 4

Ingredients:

- 1-pound cauliflower, cut into medium-sized florets
- 1 cup tomato sauce
- ½ cup of water
- 1 tablespoon tomato paste
- 1 medium white onion, diced
- 2 red bell peppers, diced
- 2 jalapeno peppers, seeded and diced
- 1 tablespoon garlic powder
- 2 teaspoons chipotle powder
- 2 teaspoons cumin
- 1 teaspoon oregano
- 1 teaspoon pepper

Directions:

1. Put the water, tomato sauce, plus tomato paste in the slow cooker. Blend. Add the spices and stir. Add the onion and peppers, and stir. Add the cauliflower and coat the cauliflower with the liquid.

2.   Cook on low for 5 hours. Once it is done, use a potato masher or blunt object to mash it until you get a rice-like consistency.

3.   Stir it well and drain any extra liquid. If you store this in the fridge, note that the cauliflower will absorb more liquid as it sits.

Nutrition:

- Calories: 205
- Fat: 18g
- Protein: 3g
- Carbs: 18g

Vegetable Ratatouille

Preparation time: 15 minutes

Cooking time: 4 hours

Servings: 6

Ingredients:

- 1 large red bell pepper, slice into squares
- 1 large eggplant, diced
- 2 large zucchinis, diced
- 1 large yellow onion, diced
- 3-2 garlic cloves, finely chopped
- 1 25-ounce jar of tomato sauce or pasta sauce
- Pinch of fresh basil

Directions:

1. Place all ingredients in the crockpot and cover with the sauce. Cook on high for 4 hours. Serve with freshly chopped basil

Nutrition:

- Calories: 215
- Fat: 18g
- Protein: 3g
- Carbs: 8g

Crockpot Parmesan Lemon Cauliflower

Preparation time: 15 minutes

Cooking time: 2 hours

Servings: 4

Ingredients :

- 1-pound cauliflower
- 2 tablespoons butter
- 2 tablespoon fresh sage or powdered
- 2 tablespoons lemon juice
- 1 cup parmesan cheese
- Parsley to garnish

Directions:

1. Place all the fixing in a bowl and thoroughly cover the cauliflower with the butter, sage, and lemon. Cook on low for 2 hours.

2. Once done, add parmesan cheese and a bit more lemon and let it steam for 10 minutes. Serve with a topping of fresh parsley.

Nutrition:

- Calories: 180
- Fat: 18g

- Protein: 3g
- Carbs: 18g

Garlic Herb Mushrooms

Preparation time: 15 minutes

Cooking time: 4 hours

Servings: 4

Ingredients:

- ¼ teaspoon thyme
- 2 bay leaves
- 1 cup vegetable broth
- ½ cup half and half
- 2 tablespoons butter
- 2 tablespoons fresh parsley, chopped
- Salt and pepper, to taste

Directions:

1. Place all of the ingredients save for the butter and the half and half in the slow cooker and put on low for 3 hours. Once done, add the butter and half for the last 15 minutes. Garnish with parsley and enjoy.

Nutrition:

- Calories: 175
- Fat: 18g
- Protein: 3g

- Carbs: 18g

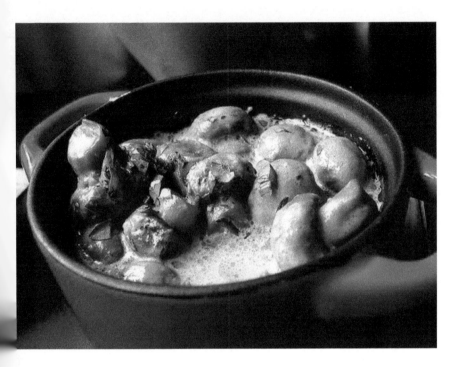

Lightning Source UK Ltd.
Milton Keynes UK
UKHW020730210621
385887UK00005B/136